Qi Gong
Meditative Postures

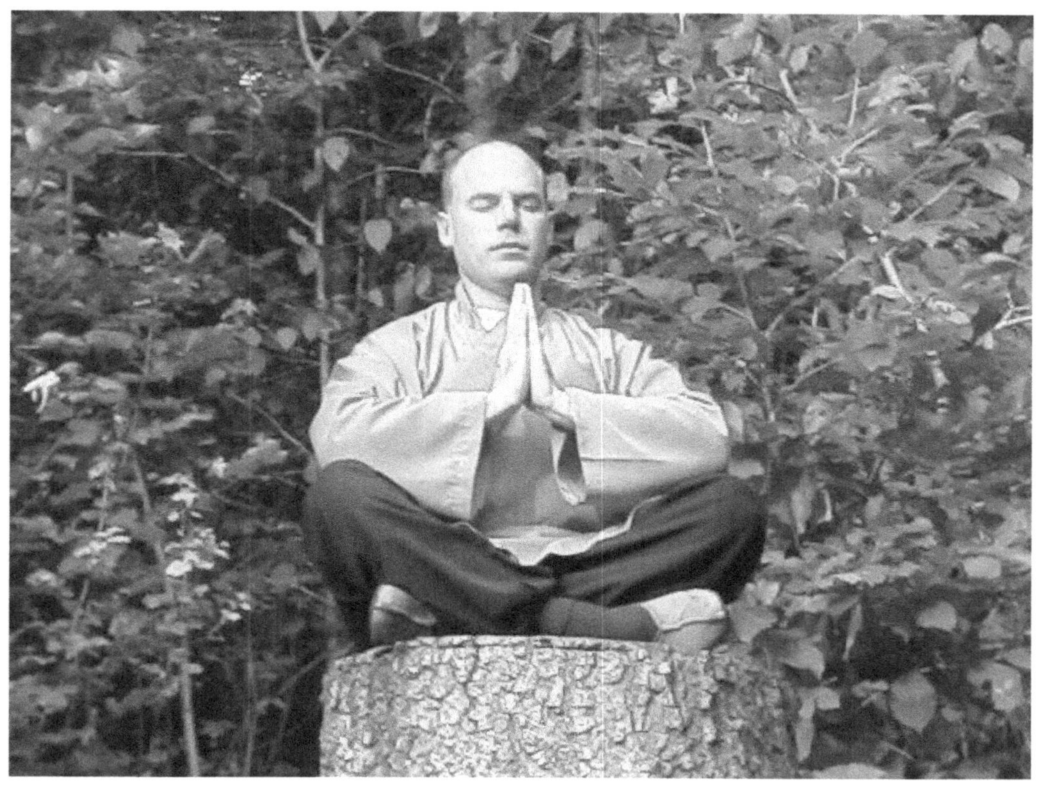

A journey of self awakening, healing, and the development of mind, body, and spirit.

Volume 1.

Al Gauthier

Important Information

Volume I. Levels 8-10

First Edition Copyright© 2021

Printed in the United States of America

Contact:

Al Gauthier

Hillside Center

8107 Laurel Bowie Rd

Bowie, MD 20715

Ph. (301)-262-1742

Facebook: Hillside Center

www.hillside.center

kuk_son1653@yahoo.com

Volume I: Levels 10-8

Volume II: Levels 7-5

Volume III: Levels 4-1

Background Information:

Mr. Al Gauthier is a martial artist and Ki Gong instructor from Bowie, MD. Mr. Gauthier has been practicing and instructing both Ki Gong and martial arts for almost half a century.

Acknowledgements:

I would like to express my gratitude and appreciation to my master's for their guidance and for opening my eyes as well as my heart to the outstanding benefits of Ki Gong.

Preface:

The objective of this training manual is to offer the individual a step by step guide to the practice of Ki Gong's meditative postures for the benefit of all humanity.

Disclaimer: This book is based on Korean Buddhist interpretations and we will use terms from the Korean language. The term Ki is used for vital energy and it is highly recommended that you learn basic Korean terms for better understanding. This book will be the first of a series on these postures and will combine the first three sets out of a ten level course.

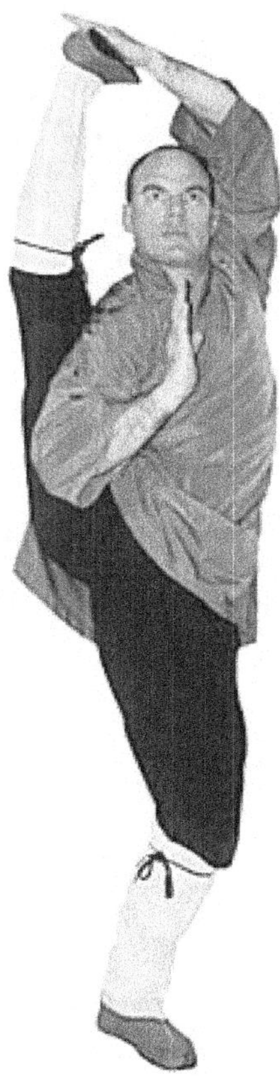

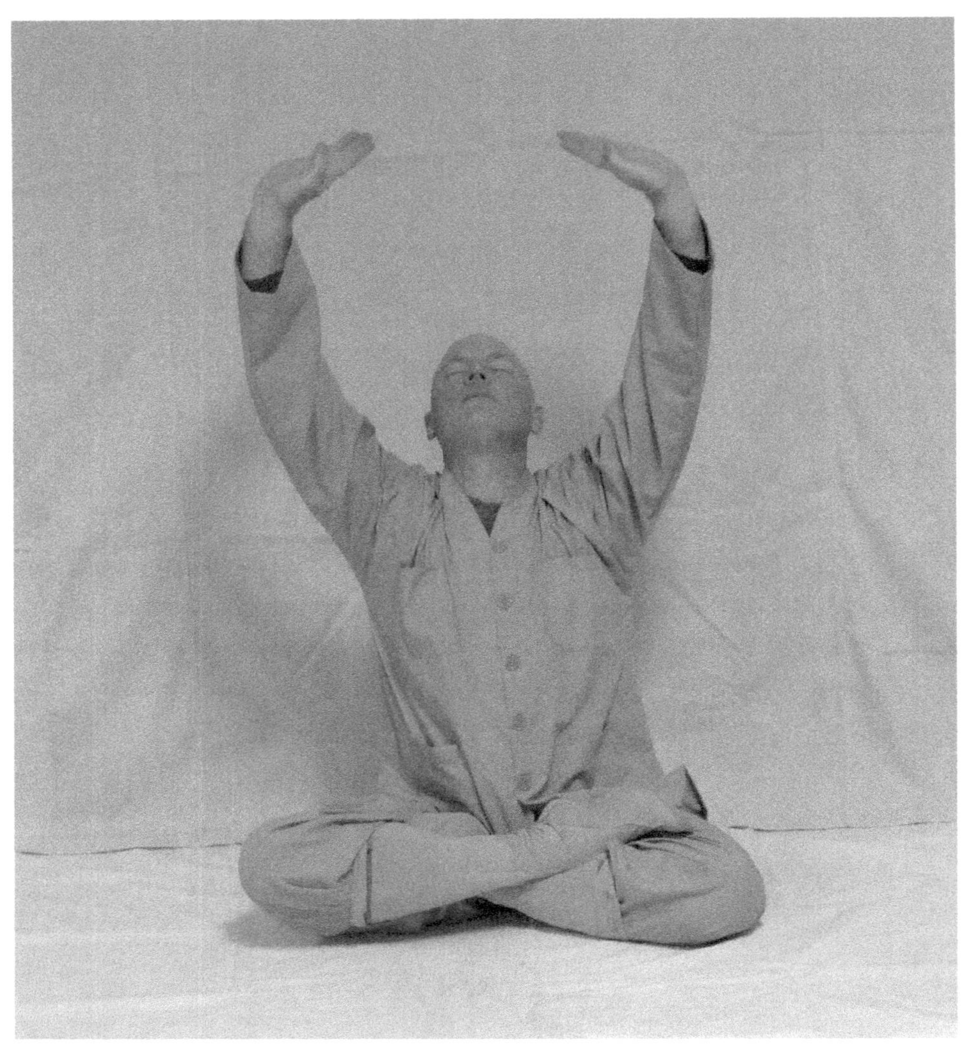

"If you look for the truth outside of yourself, it gets further and further away. Yet When you achieve that perfect harmony of mind and body, and can control your Qi, the result is a great spiritual awakening..." - Master Tung Shen - 9th Century Philosopher

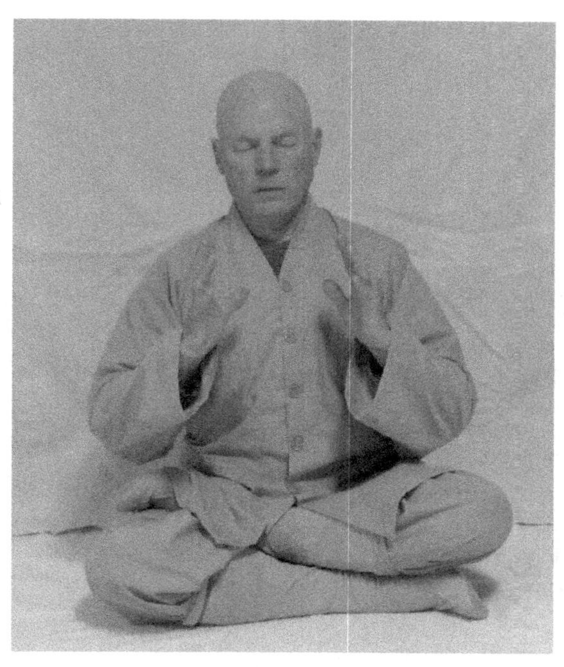

Chapter I: Introduction

What is Qi Gong (Ki Gong)?

Ki Gong is an ancient system of exercise that cultivates and improves the health of those that practice it, both mentally, physically, and spiritually. It places an emphasis on breathing to collect Ki (vital energy) and a systematic practice with development (Gong). This body of knowledge is vast and varied, all of which comes from thousands of years of practice from a variety of Asian countries such as Tibet, India, China, Korea and Japan. This practice is inseparable from the lifestyles of both Buddhist and Taoist Monks.

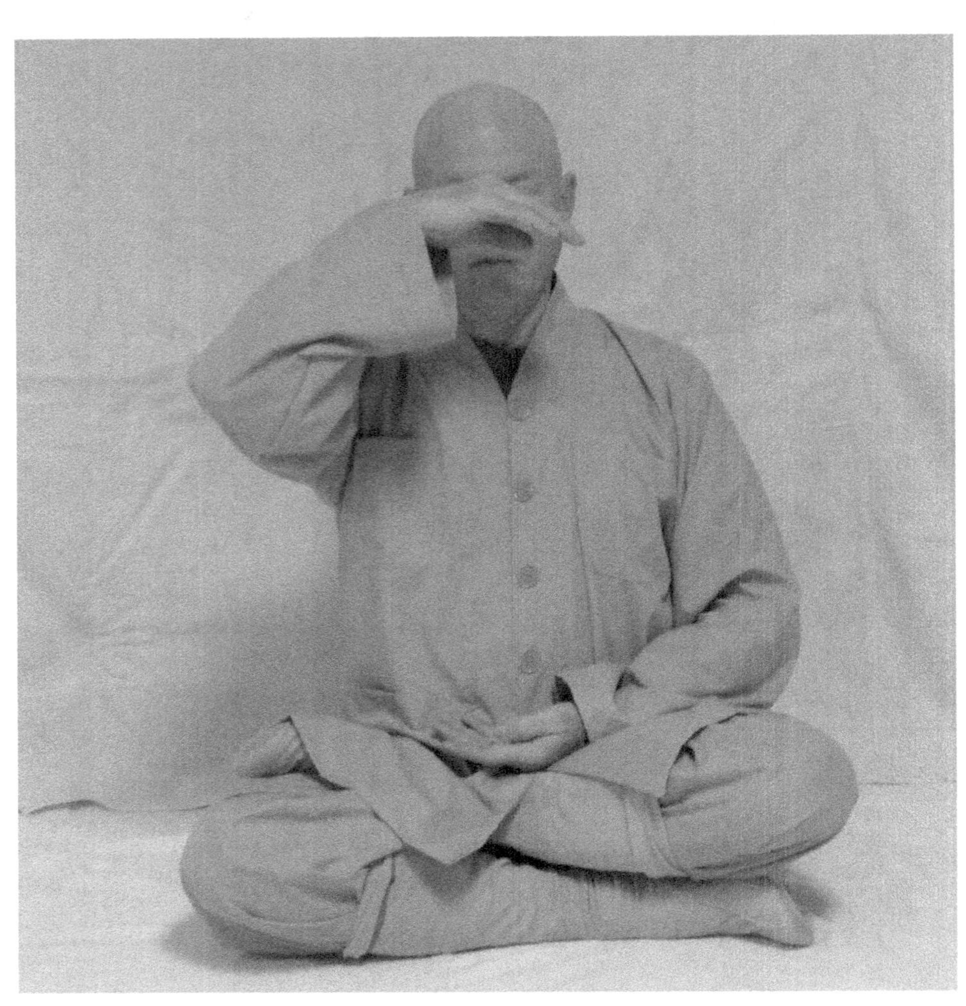

Chapter II

"The life force is very real; at its center appears truth" - Lao Tzu

What are meditative postures?

Meditative postures (Haeng Gong) are designed to be used with meditation to tonify or sedate (Ki) energy and promote its circulation through the energy system while accumulating this energy in your lower abdomen area. Each meditation practice set or level has a unique purpose and formula. The mind plays an active role with intent, focus, and visualization. After the correct posture has been achieved, it will become a subconscious process. These sets follow a prescribed doctrine, which helps the student understand what they may experience during this process. It can be life altering and extremely profound. Once secluded in religious monasteries in the far east this has become widely available for the west. We are truly blessed to have this knowledge and wisdom in our times. The practitioner embarks on a personal journey. The first step is to become awoken and validate the process then there is a type of rebirth and self healing on a physical and emotional level. There comes a point in the journey where there can be a great spiritual awakening and enlightenment.

Let's get started...

Find a quiet place that is warm and peaceful. Soft music, incense, and candles can help facilitate relaxation creating a calm, tranquil feeling. These steps are conducive to this practice.

Haeng Gong Level 10

The sets go from beginner level 10 to the highest level 1.

Haeng Gong practice should begin after you have relaxed and completed an energy wash in the (corpse posture). Visualize and guide Ki energy through your body starting at your head to your toes. You will become aware of Ki while learning to relax and also reduce your stress.

First posture (Il Ban)

Objective: Relaxation, stress reduction, Dan Jun activation

1. Form a heart shape at your navel and practice lower (Dan Jun) breathing. Inhale to your Dan Jun - hold - exhale out of the nose and relax. Repeat the process. Do not force it. Exhalations should be slightly longer than the inhalation. After practicing for about ten minutes slowly turn to your right side and sit cross legged in preparation for sitting meditation.

<u>**What is Un Ki Shim Gong?**</u>

This is a seated meditation where you will use your mind to direct the flow of Ki at the hands. During this process, you will activate powerful points in the body such as the points in the palms and the point on the top of your head. The movement of the hands are graceful and should become an unconscious movement flowing from the Ki flow. You may feel heat between the hands or the sensation of two magnets pushing against each other. It helps validate the existence of Ki energy.

Inhale and spread your palms apart. Exhale and bring your palms together without touching. Repeat like an ocean wave.

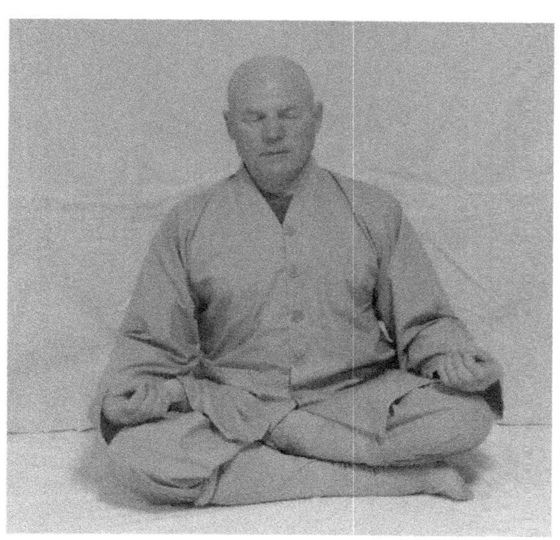

Preparation with thumb and first two fingers together

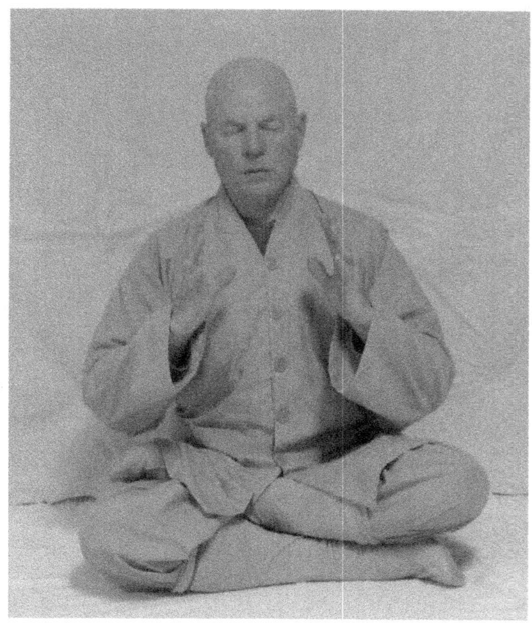

Bring your palms in front of your chest

After practicing for about five minutes return to your starting position with your hands on your knees.

Note: Un Ki Shim Gong helps you develop a Ki connection at your hands for personal energy wash and healing others.

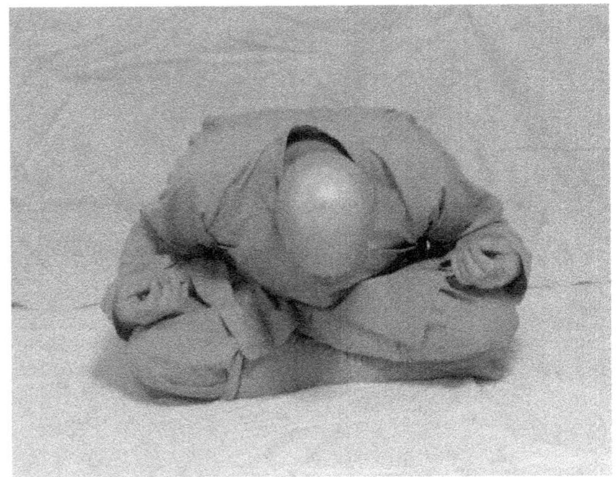

Closing - Inhale to the Dan Jun and then exhale through your mouth. Next inhale through the nose and then exhale through the teeth while bending forward. Repeat this twice.

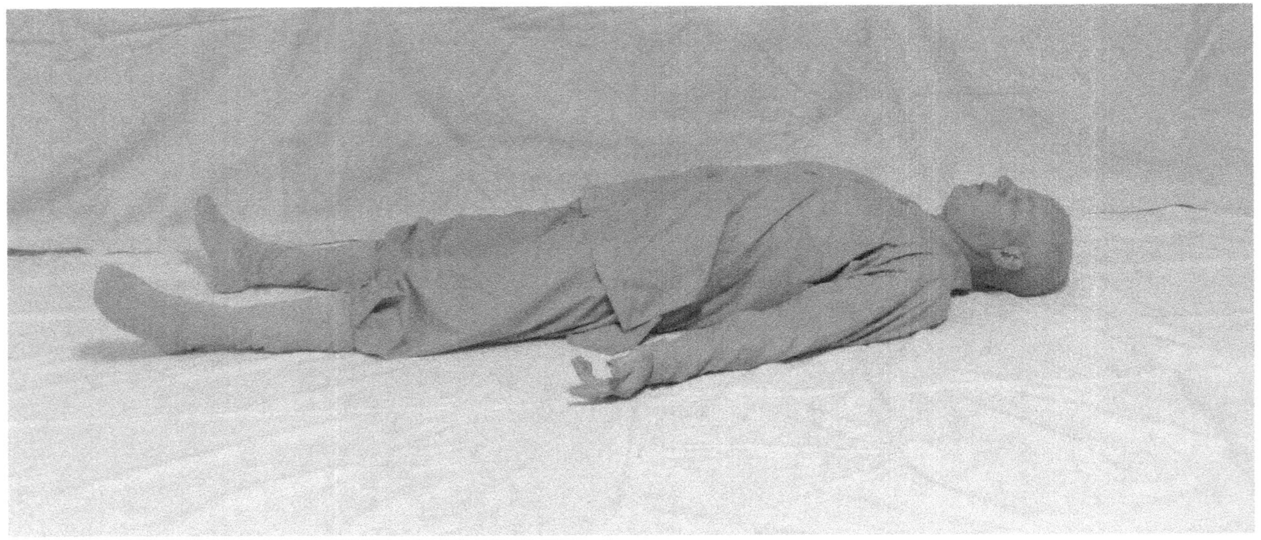

End your Haeng Gong practice by laying back in the corpse posture and rest for a minute. After resting, rub your palms together making them warm. Cover your open eyes and send Ki to them and rotate your eyes, Next, rub your face, scalp, chest, abdomen and Dan Jun. Stretch your body and you can also perform gentle floor stretches.

Turn to your right side and stand back up. You can also transition to a kneeling posture and perform some Dan Jun breathing before standing back up.

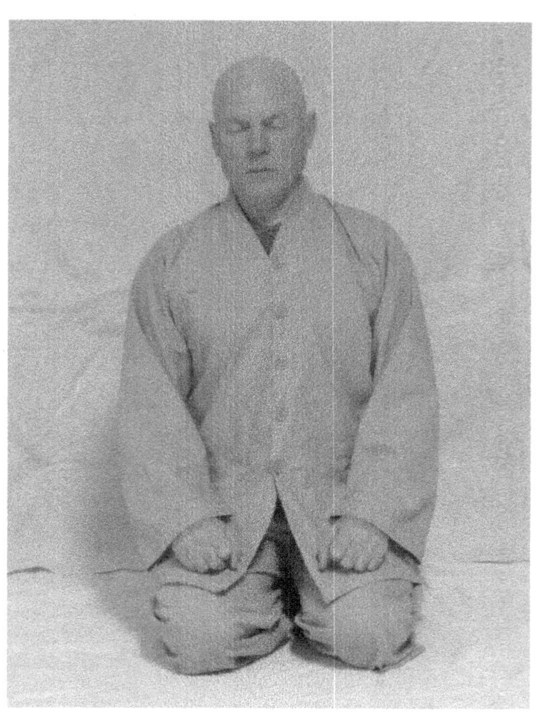

<u>**Conclusion:**</u>

For some the first experience of Ki energy can be very moving and some may experience tears of joy. We are awoken to a great divine cosmic energy. This feeling and connection can be incredible.

You should practice this level for one month before advancing to level 9.

Haeng Gong Level 9 (Ku Gup)

Objective: Ki accumulation - relaxation

Repeat the corpse posture with body washes before starting the first posture. For the following 9 levels there will be five postures and one Un Ki Shim Gong posture. Level 9 will consist of a tonification and sedation process as we open up our meridian system. We will promote Ki flow and cultivation in the Dan Jun. We will also activate the acupoints in the feet. You should breathe in through these points to the Dan Jun then exhale back out through these points for the first three postures.

Note: Hold each posture for 2 - 3 minutes

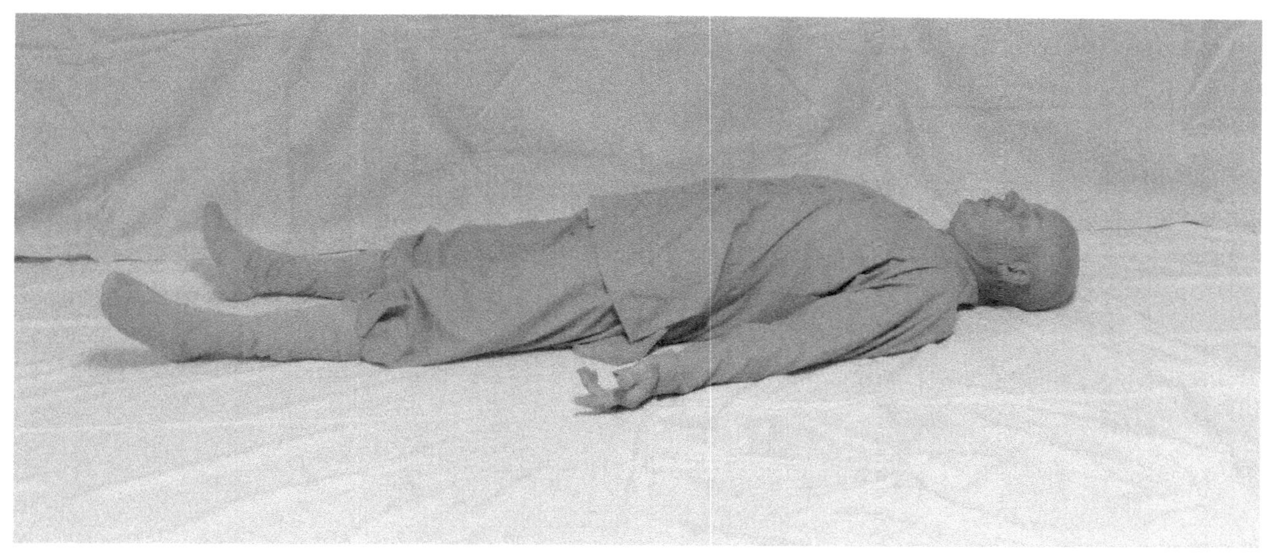

Haeng Gong Level 9 Postures

Lying Posture (Wa Gong)

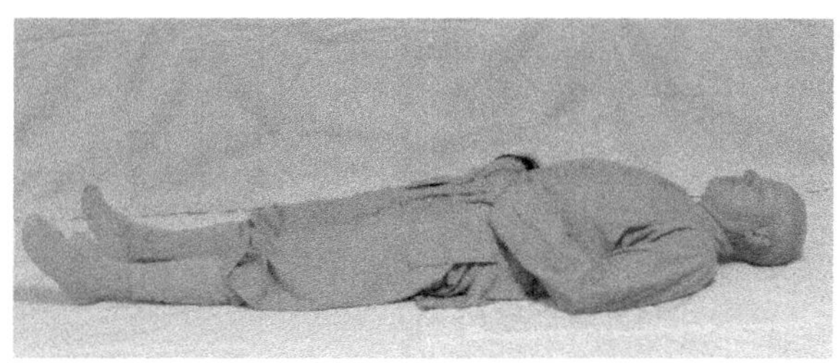

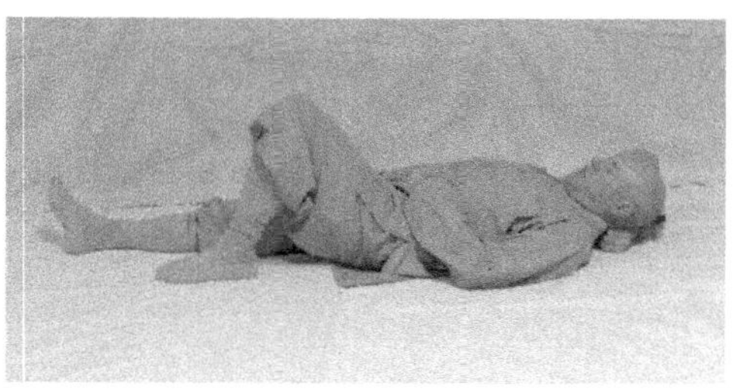

1. Il Ban

2. Ee Ban

Note: Support neck with thumb tucked inside fist.

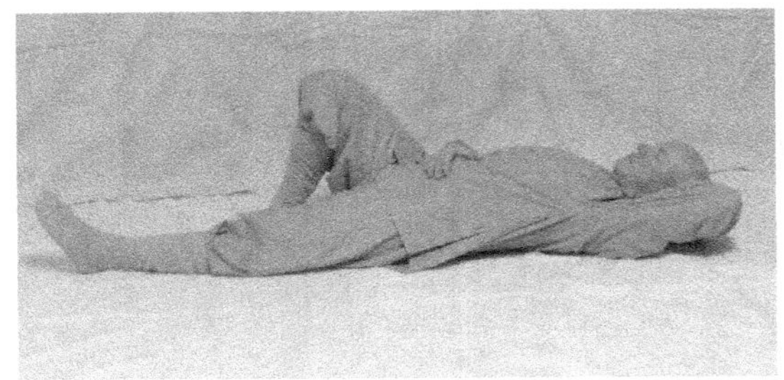

3. Sahm Ban

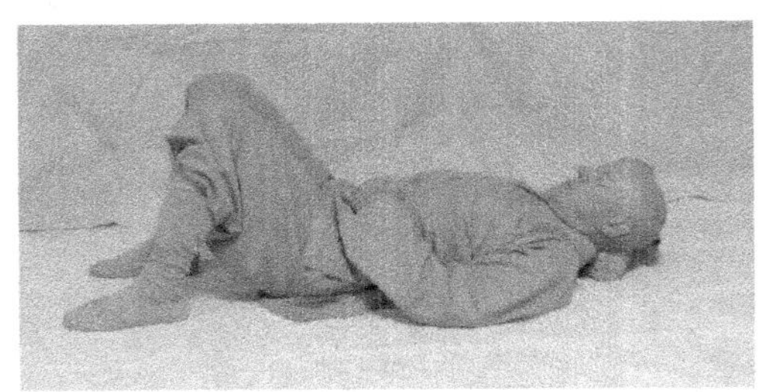

4. Sa Ban

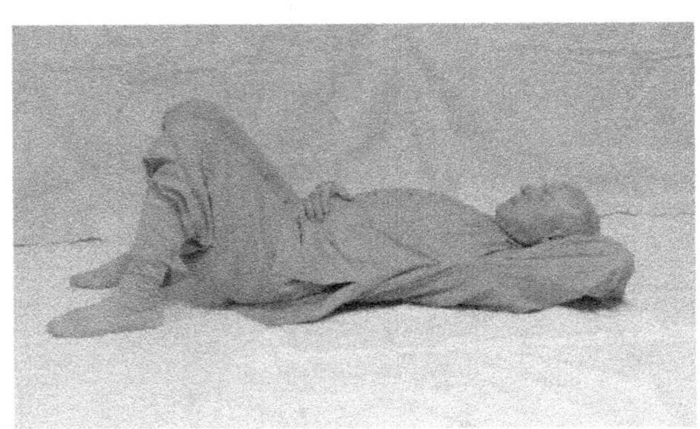

5. Oh Ban

For postures 4 and 5, practice normal Dan Jun breathing.

Next, straighten your legs, turn to your right side and be seated cross legged for seated meditation.

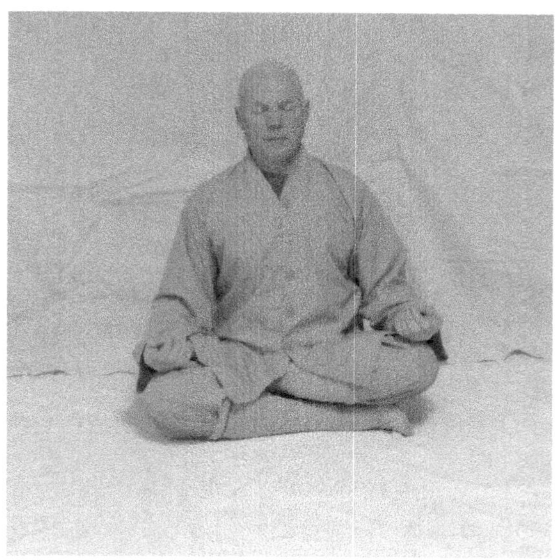

Start from a cross legged preparatory posture

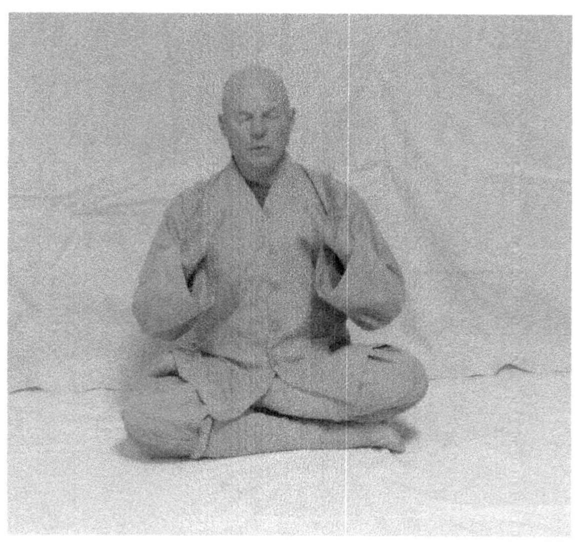

Perform Un Ki Shim Gong as in level 10.

Practice for about 5 minutes and then return to preparatory posture. Now, lie back and rest for a minute.

Refer to the wake up exercise in level 10 before standing back up. You should practice this set daily for about one to two months. You may now be feeling

1 warmth in Dan Jun and hands. You may also develop a sweet tasting saliva.
When you do, swallow in three gulps sending it to Dan Jun.

Haeng Gong Level Eight (Pahl Gup)

Objective: Improve the function of internal organs and Ki accumulation.

Level eight Haeng Gong is the most physically demanding, up to date. It can be very difficult to hold the postures at first. As you master the flow through your acupoints (yong chon) you will experience a feeling of strength and lightness. Your form is maintained through your Ki flow. It is quite remarkable. This set is one of the greatest Ki Gong sets that you can practice. It is a landmark and can be life changing as you cultivate your mind, body and spirit during this practice.

Preparation will be the same as in the other Haeng Gong sets.

Notes: For this set, we activate our Yong Chon, Jang Shim and Myung Moon points. The Myung Moon point is remarkable because of its proximity to the Dan Jun. Hold each posture for two to three minutes. Practice this set daily for about three months.

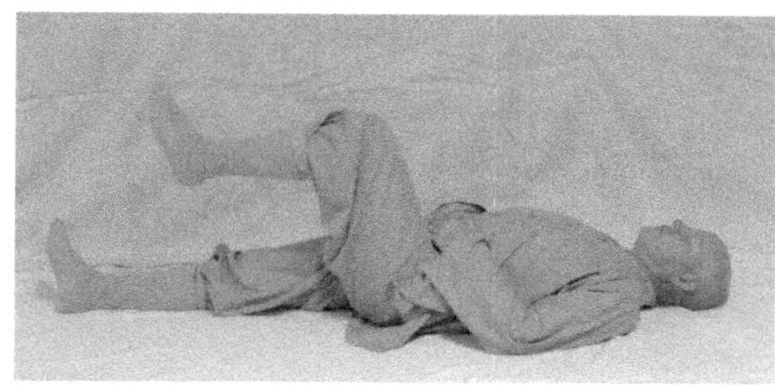

1. Il Ban - Yong Chon Breathing

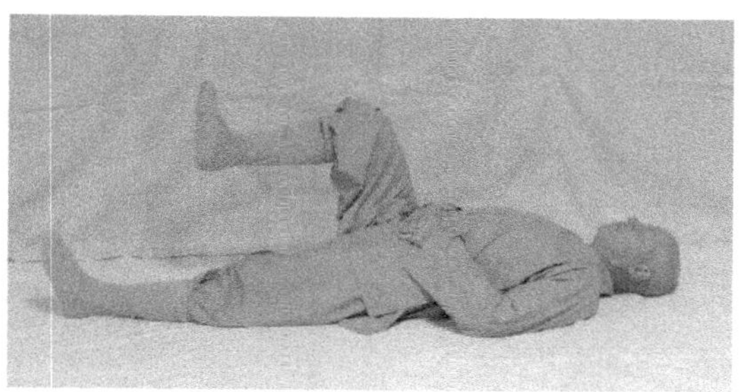

2. Ee Ban

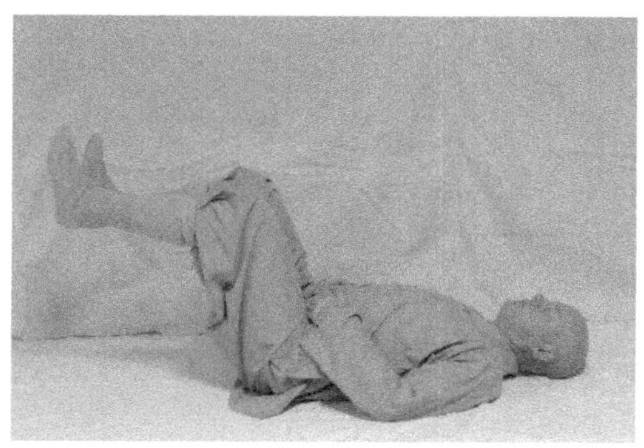

3. Sahm Ban

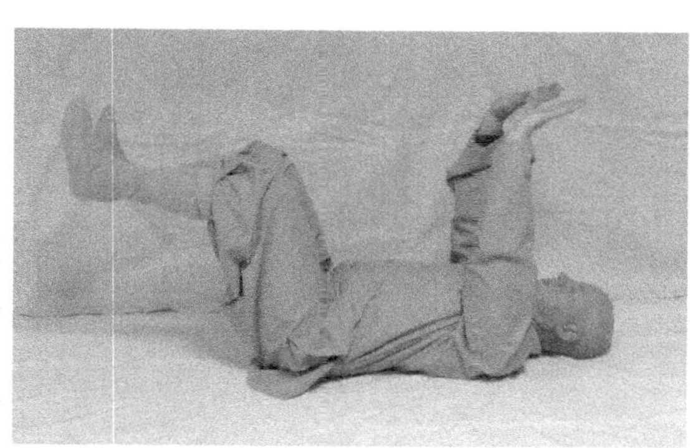

4. Sa Ban

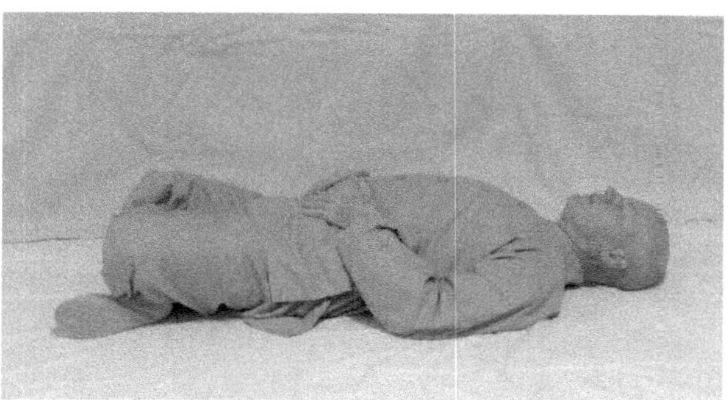

5. Oh Ban

Activate Myung Moon breathing - (spirit gate)

Note: Inhale through points to Dan Jun and exhale back out through points.

Level 8

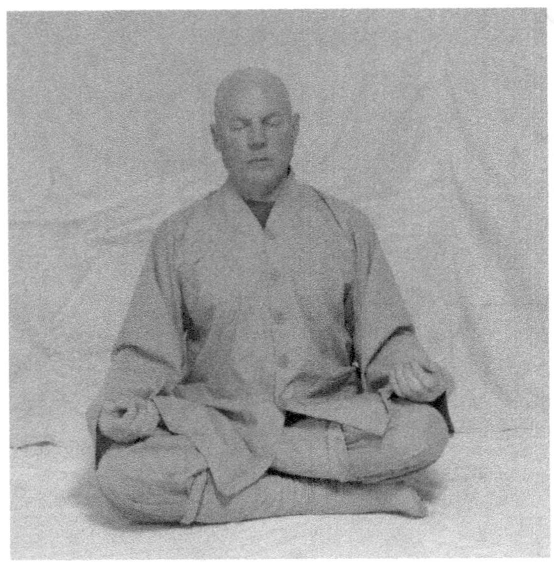

Preparatory Posture

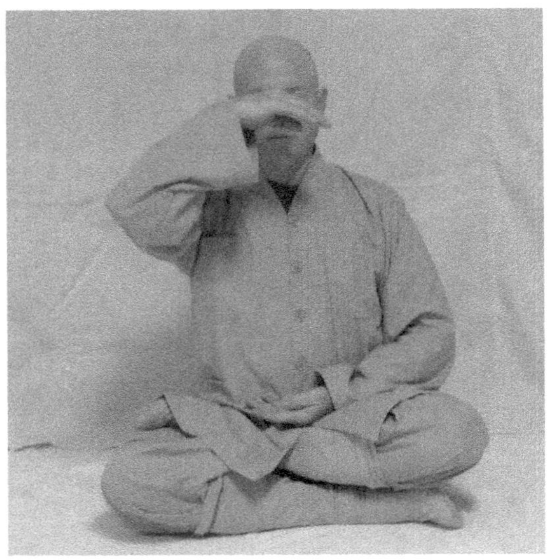

Perform raising and lowering palm (15) times and then switch hands.

Practice for about 5 minutes and then close as in previous sets.

General Notes:

Haeng Gong practice is a great compliment to the energy arts like yoga and the martial arts. We encourage you to keep a journal of your progress.

Have your health and energy levels improved?

Are you more patient and peaceful?

Are you feeling heat or energy in your hands?

Be honest and objective.

Typically, Haeng Gong is used at the end of a class. You should feel relaxed and energized with a feeling of calm aliveness.

Haeng Gong helps you to live in the present moment.

Enjoy your journey in health and happiness. It is a new frontier of amazing discoveries and self realization.

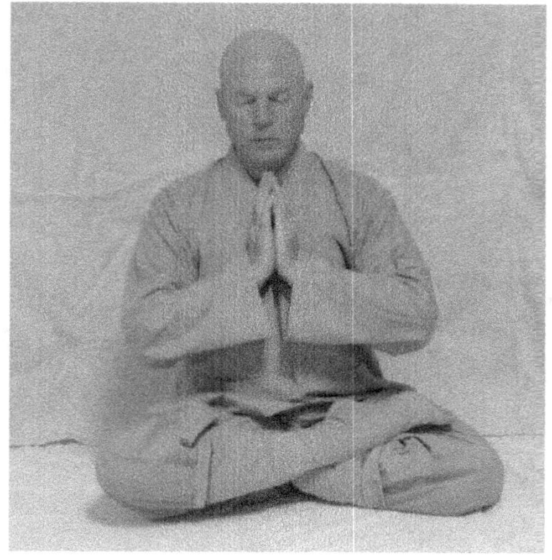

<u>**Haeng Gong Doctrine:**</u>

      The ancients have given us their teachings. They tell us that if we follow their lessons that we will experience many new and incredible things. As an experienced practitioner of these doctrines, I can tell you that they are true and very real. They were life changing for me. What is ancient becomes new. We wake up to this divine energy and we embrace it. We sleep better and feel better. We have a heightened sense of self and others. We are healing physically, mentally and spiritually. We feel connected to humanity and our source. Our posture is corrected and we become more flexible. We will detox and purify our bodies, particularly our immune system which includes the function of all our internal organs. Every Haeng Gong is an exciting experience and treasure. Enjoy your journey…

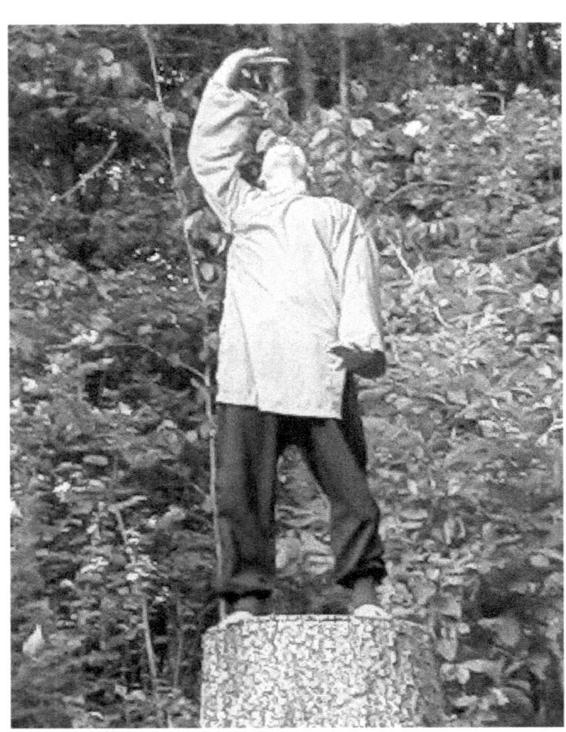

Words of wisdom

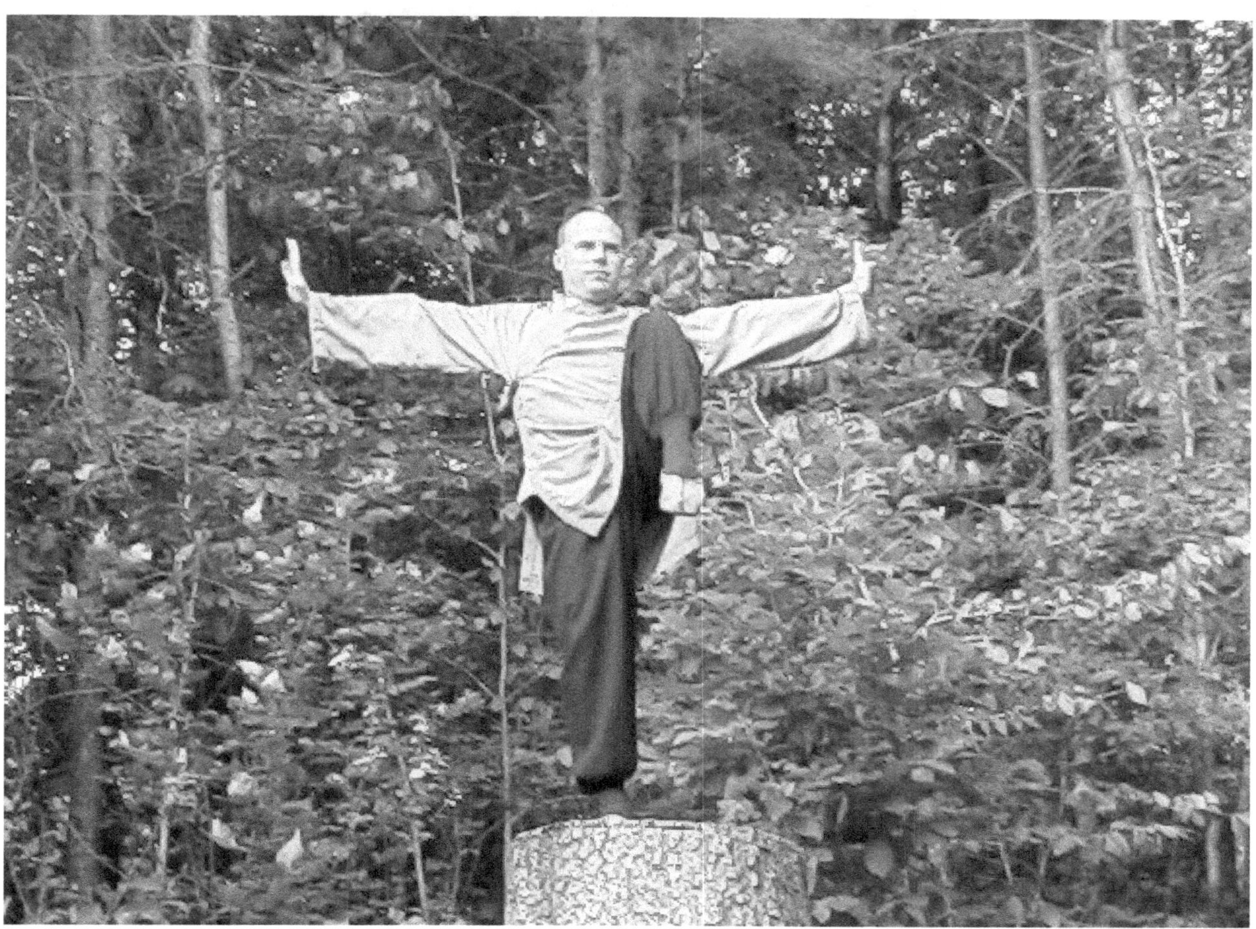

"Having mastered the body through the ancient teachings so that it becomes a fit habitation for the soul; Having the senses, emotions, and mind under control. The master discards the worn-out sheaths of desire, fear and confusion and passes into the state of enlightenment and freedom."

Ancient sage…

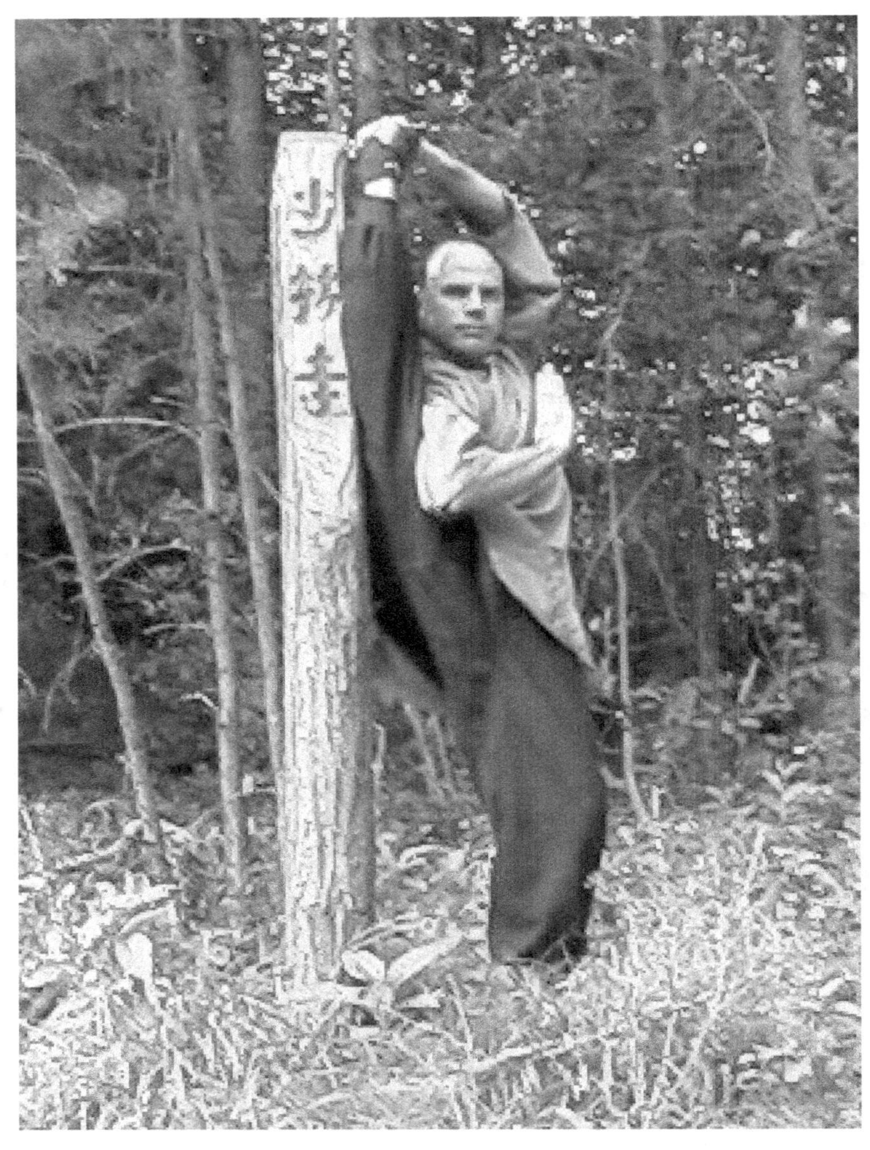

"The soft and the yielding overcome the rigid and hard but few people put this into practice".

The Tao Te Ching

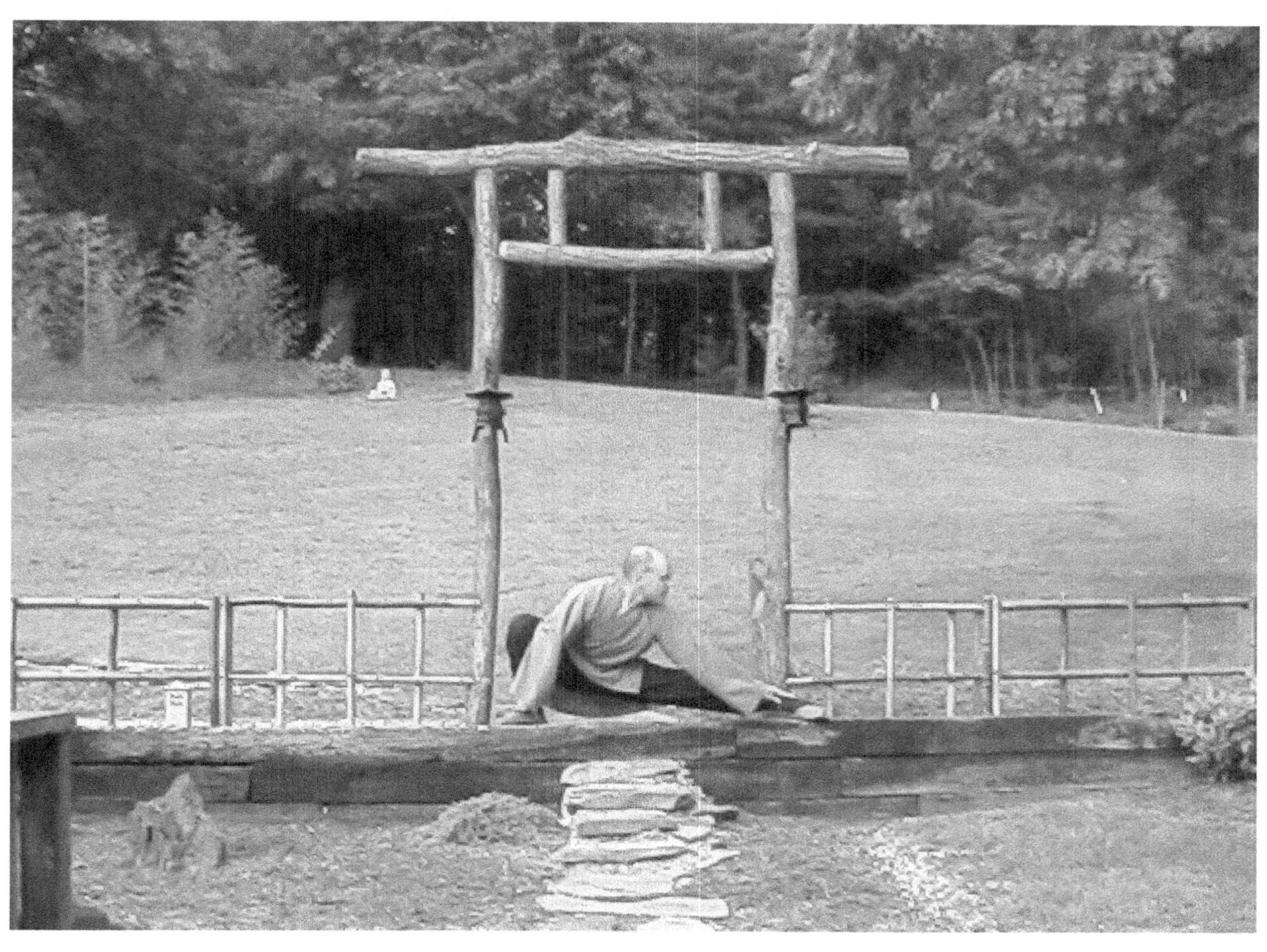

"What you think you become. What you feel, you attract. What you imagine you create."

Buddha

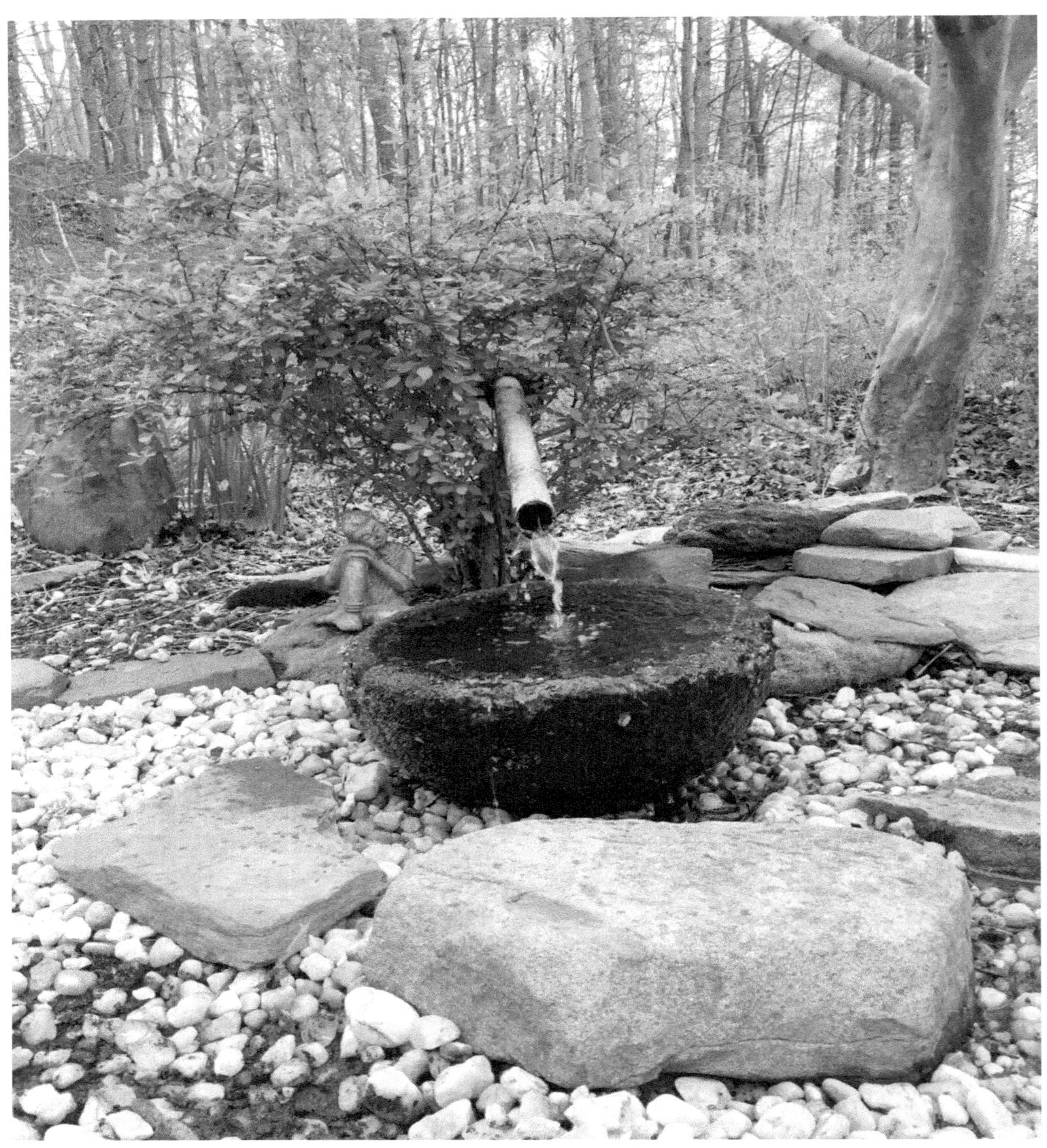

"Water is fluid, soft, and yielding. But water will wear away the rock, which is rigid and cannot yield. As a rule, whatever is soft and yielding will overcome whatever is rigid and hard. This is another paradox: what is soft is strong".

Lao Tzu

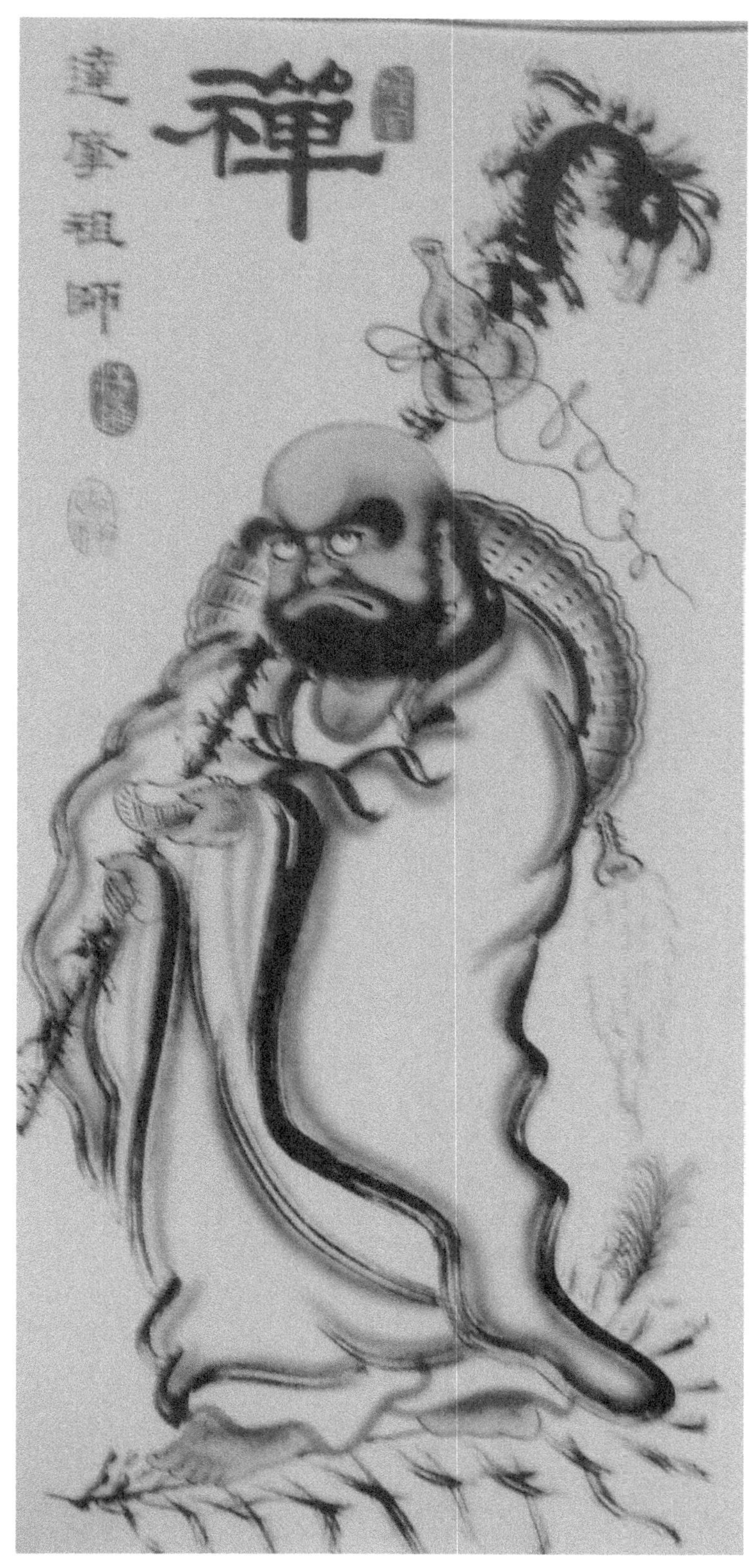

"The essence of the way is detachment."

Bodhidharma